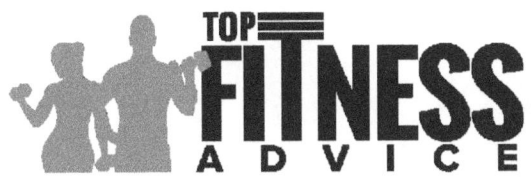

KETOGENIC DIET

A Beginner's Guide PLUS 35 Recipes to Kick Start Your Weight Loss, Boost Energy, and Slim Down FAST!

LINDA WESTWOOD

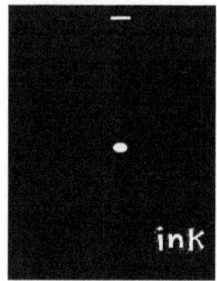

First published in 2016 by Venture Ink Publishing

Copyright © Top Fitness Advice 2019

All rights reserved.

No part of this book may be reproduced in any form without permission in writing from the author. No part of this publication may be reproduced or transmitted in any form or by any means, mechanic, electronic, photocopying, recording, by any storage or retrieval system, or transmitted by email without the permission in writing from the author and publisher.

Requests to the publisher for permission should be addressed to publishing@ventureink.co

For more information about the contents of this book or questions to the author, please contact Linda Westwood at linda@topfitnessadvice.com

Disclaimer

This book provides wellness management information in an informative and educational manner only, with information that is general in nature and that is not specific to you, the reader. The contents of this book are intended to assist you and other readers in your personal wellness efforts. Consult your physician regarding the applicability of any information provided in this book to you.

Nothing in this book should be construed as personal advice or diagnosis, and must not be used in this manner. The information provided about conditions is general in nature. This information does not cover all possible uses, actions, precautions, side-effects, or interactions of medicines, or medical procedures. The information in this book should not be considered as complete and does not cover all diseases, ailments, physical conditions, or their treatment.

You should consult with your physician before beginning any exercise, weight loss, or health care program. This book should not be used in place of a call or visit to a competent health-care professional. You should consult a health care professional before adopting any of the suggestions in this book or before drawing inferences from it.

Any decision regarding treatment and medication for your condition should be made with the advice and consultation of a qualified health care professional. If you have, or suspect you have, a health-care problem, then you should immediately contact a qualified health care professional for treatment.

No Warranties: The author and publisher don't guarantee or warrant the quality, accuracy, completeness, timeliness, appropriateness or suitability of the information in this book, or of any product or services referenced in this book.

The information in this book is provided on an "as is" basis and the author and publisher make no representations or warranties of any kind with respect to this information. This book may contain inaccuracies, typographical errors, or other errors.

Liability Disclaimer: The publisher, author, and other parties involved in the creation, production, provision of information, or delivery of this book specifically disclaim any responsibility, and shall not be held liable for any damages, claims, injuries, losses, liabilities, costs, or obligations including any direct, indirect, special, incidental, or consequences damages (collectively known as "Damages") whatsoever and howsoever caused, arising out of, or in connection with the use or misuse of the site and the information contained within it, whether such Damages arise in contract, tort, negligence, equity, statute law, or by way of other legal theory.

Table of Contents

Disclaimer	3
Who is this book for?	7
What will this book teach you?	9
Chapter 1: How Your Body Gains Weight, and Why It's So Hard to Lose	11
Chapter 2: How the Ketogenic Diet Works	17
Chapter 3: Other Benefits of the Ketogenic Diet	19
Chapter 4: The Basics of the Ketogenic Diet	23
Chapter 5: Safely Following the Ketogenic Diet	27
Ketogenic Meal Plan Recipes	33
Conclusion	101
Final Words	103

Would you prefer to listen to my book, rather than read it?

Download the audiobook version for free!

If you go to the special link below and sign up to Audible as a new customer, you can get the audiobook version of my book completely free.

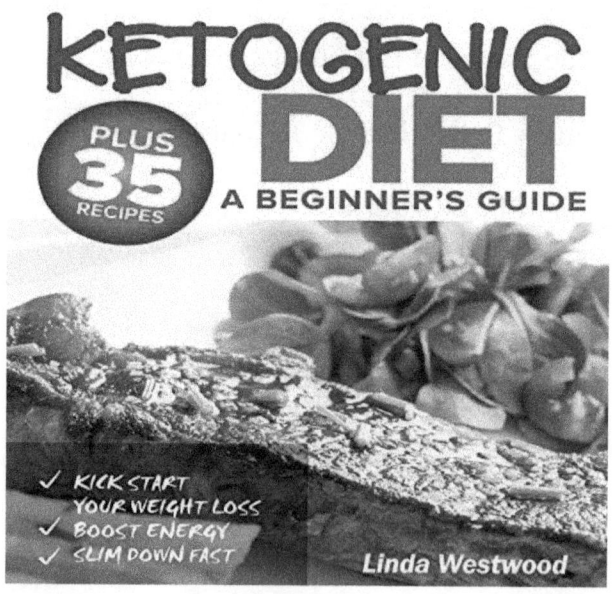

Go here to get your audiobook version for free:

TopFitnessAdvice.com/go/ketogenic

Who is this book for?

Are you someone who is faithful to your workout routine and who honestly tries to watch what you eat and how much, but still finds it hard to lose weight and keep it off?

Do you find that every diet plan and every meal plan you ever try only leaves you hungry and unsatisfied, overwhelmed with cravings, and unhappy with everything on your plate?

Do you get fatigued in between meals, and find yourself reaching for a snack just for a quick boost of energy?

If all of this sounds familiar, then **this book is for you!**

The ketogenic diet is not just another starvation diet that has you eating unappetizing foods in tiny portions, but it works with the body's metabolism to turn it into a real fat burning machine.

Many professional athletes and bodybuilders follow a ketogenic diet, to burn their fat stores and keep off unwanted fat while turning up the furnace of their body's muscles, so they become lean and toned in no time.

With the ketogenic diet, you don't need to actually weigh and measure food, and can fill up on healthy and delicious choices so you never walk away from the table feeling hungry and dissatisfied again!

You can see pounds and inches being shed within the first few days of following a ketogenic diet, and for many people, their cholesterol levels drop while their energy levels rise.

If you're ready to get started with an eating plan that keeps you full while helping you shed the weight, let's first explain some basics about the diet and the eating plan, how it works, how it can benefit you, and how you can try easy and delicious recipes right in your own kitchen.

What will this book teach you?

To successfully follow any diet or eating plan, it's good to know how the body works, how and why you gain weight, and how to keep yourself safe while shedding those extra pounds. In this book, we'll cover all of that, and so much more!

In these pages, you'll learn the basics of how your body actually gets the energy you need for everyday activities, as well as why you often get tired and fatigued when you try to lose weight.

You'll also learn the real reason why simply restricting your calorie intake or eating less food is often not the right choice for weight loss, or the healthiest.

Of course, knowing the wrong thing to do when you want to shed pounds and keep them off for good is only half the equation. We'll also discuss why and how the ketogenic diet works, and how to follow it properly so you get good results while staying healthy.

We'll also share some of our favorite recipes and cooking tips for staying on the ketogenic diet and finally shedding pounds without ever feeling hungry or deprived.

If you're ready to learn what you need to know about the ketogenic diet and are ready to start losing weight and gaining muscle tone, let's first talk about the body and weight loss, and how the ketogenic diet can help.

Chapter 1

How Your Body Gains Weight, and Why It's So Hard to Lose

To understand why and how the ketogenic diet works for successful weight loss, it's good to first understand some basics about how the body works when it comes to weight gain.

Your body's weight is a balance between calories consumed and calories burned; if you eat more calories than you need for physical activity, your body converts these unused calories into fat.

This fat is held by your body as an energy reserve, in case your calorie consumption drops and you don't consume enough for the energy you need. This is why diets that severely restrict your calorie intake may work for weight loss, but of course they're also very difficult to follow!

Restricting your calorie intake leads to hunger pains, cravings, low blood sugar, and fatigue, since you're not giving your body the calories it's accustomed to; in turn, your energy levels drop.

The hunger you feel when you greatly restrict your calories can also interfere with healthy weight loss. This is because you may get so hungry that you decide to grab a snack between meals, and don't realize how many calories you're adding to your daily intake.

You may think you've limited your calories for the day, but that snack might add several hundred calories to your daily diet. Your overwhelming hunger can also cause you to overeat at a meal, because you're so eager to get some food into your stomach!

Even with the best of intentions and strongest resolve, trying to severely limit your calorie intake can actually have the opposite effect of having you lose weight; you may simply gain weight because you wind up consuming more calories through snacking and overeating, versus losing those unwanted pounds.

Another problem with these types of eating plans is that, when you stop giving your body the calories it needs for energy, your system also turns to its own muscles for energy.

The body will use the protein and amino acids in these muscles for energy, causing them to get weaker. This includes the heart, as the heart is also a muscle! As a matter of fact, it's not unusual for someone suffering from conditions like anorexia or bulimia, or who is always following a severely restrictive diet, to see long-term or even permanent damage to their heart.

Another reason it's so difficult to burn off this stored fat is that the body uses the glucose it gets from food you eat for immediate energy. This glucose is mostly concentrated in carbohydrates and sugars, but is also found in many forms of protein and other such foods. As long as the body has this steady supply of glucose from food, it won't need to turn to your fat stores for energy.

This is where the ketogenic diet comes into play. Following this eating plan means reducing the amount of glucose you are giving your body so that it must burn fat for energy. In turn, the pounds melt away and you're able to keep them off for good, without starving.

Let's take a closer look at the ketogenic diet itself so you can learn more about how it works and how it can help you reach your weight loss goals, while helping you build strong, lean muscles.

Discover Scientifically-Proven "Shortcuts" & "Hacks" to Lose Weight FASTER (With Very Little Effort)

For this month only, you can get Linda's best-selling & most popular book absolutely free – *Weight Loss Secrets You NEED to Know*.

Get Your FREE Copy Here:
TopFitnessAdvice.com/Bonus

Discover scientifically-proven tips to help you lose weight faster and easier than ever before. With this book, readers were able to improve their weight loss results and fitness levels. So, it's highly recommended that you get this book, especially while it's free!

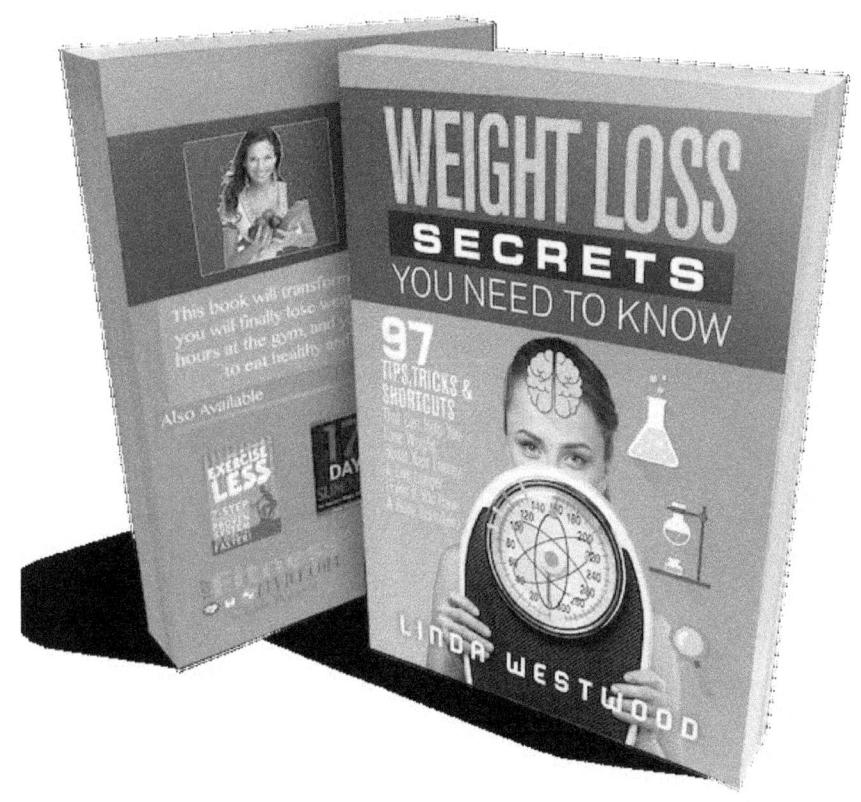

Get Your FREE Copy Here:
TopFitnessAdvice.com/Bonus

Chapter 2

How the Ketogenic Diet Works

Now that you know a little something about how the body works with the foods you eat and how your system converts food into either energy or stored fat, let's take a closer look at the ketogenic diet or eating plan in particular.

It's good to know, not just how it works, but why it's different than other eating plans as well as how and why it's safe for weight loss and for building muscle.

Reducing Glucose Intake

If your body normally uses the glucose it gets from food for energy, and you want it to start using your fat stores instead, it would seem obvious that you need to stop feeding your body so much glucose in the first place!

A ketogenic diet greatly reduces your glucose intake by reducing the amount of carbohydrates you get from food, mostly from baked goods like bread, as well as from pasta and cereals. This glucose is also very abundant in fruit and natural sweeteners like honey, and of course pure sugar.

Foods like vegetables and protein have a very low amount of glucose, so they're not as restricted on the ketogenic diet. Fats like dairy products and oils have little to no glucose, so they may make up the bulk of your ketogenic diet.

When your body is not getting its standard supply of glucose from what you're eating, it will have no choice but to turn to its stores of fat for energy. This is what's called the metabolic state of ketosis. Your body uses fatty acids, called ketones, for energy, burning up that fat in the process.

Maintaining Protein and Fat Intake

Because the ketogenic diet doesn't mean just restricting calories and because it also allows for lots of protein, your body won't start to use up the protein and amino acids in your muscles for energy during this ketosis stage.

The calories you get from the protein you're allowed, along with sufficient amounts of fat, will keep you energized and not make you feel hungry. The fat you eat with the ketogenic diet will also mean protecting your heart, circulatory system, and so much else, as these need healthy fats to stay hydrated and healthy.

I hope that you are enjoying this book so far, and if you could spare 30 seconds, I would greatly appreciate you leaving a review on Amazon.com.

Chapter 3

Other Benefits of the Ketogenic Diet

When you are able to turn your body into a true fat burning machine, you may see your extra pounds melt away quickly and easily, even without ever stepping foot in the gym. This itself is one of the best things about following the ketogenic diet!

However, would you be surprised to learn that there are other benefits to the ketogenic diet, making it one of the best you can follow even if you're not trying to lose weight? Let's consider some of those here.

Steady Energy

When your body is using the glucose from foods that you eat for energy, you may see that your energy levels rise and fall throughout the day, according to your meals. After eating, your body has that immediate burst of energy since it has its needed supply of glucose.

However, once that glucose is used up, your energy levels fall, as your body is not yet trained to turn to fat stores or any other energy source.

Once you train your body to rely on your own fat stores for energy and not this intermittent supply of glucose, your energy levels then also level off and become more even throughout the day.

Rather than getting sluggish in the afternoon or an hour after dinner, you may find that you have consistent energy no matter the time of day and no matter your schedule of meals.

Triglycerides

Triglycerides are fat molecules that are found in the blood, and they're a strong indication or risk factor for heart disease and other heart-related health conditions.

When you follow the ketogenic diet and your body starts burning fat for energy, your levels of triglycerides usually drop. In turn, you may actually lower your risk of a heart attack and heart disease.

Controlling Blood Sugar Levels

The glucose in carbs will find their way into the bloodstream, spiking your blood sugar levels. There are some dangers to this; for one thing, your body needs to produce insulin from the pancreas to break down that sugar.

Consistently working the pancreas in this way can eventually cause it to "malfunction" and not produce enough insulin, or produce none at all, and this leads to diabetes.

That glucose can also interfere with proper blood circulation so that your organs don't get the blood they need for repairing and restoring themselves; many diabetics have vision problems or failing kidneys because of how organs are affected.

However, by reducing the amount of glucose in the bloodstream by reducing the carbohydrates and sugars you eat, your risk factors for diabetes are reduced and, in some cases, the condition is even reversed!

Brain Health

Many people tend to forget that the brain is an organ and, like all other organs in the body, it needs to be nourished properly in order to work properly.

If you have too much glucose in your blood so that it interrupts healthy blood flow, this includes the blood that goes to the brain! Without this healthy, nourishing blood, the tissue of the brain itself may begin to break down and not be repaired and restored. In turn, brain function, including memory, concentration, focus, and problem solving, can all suffer.

The healthy oils you fill up on with a ketogenic diet are also used by the brain to protect its own tissue. There is a thin coating over the brain that is needed for the electrical impulses and connection that create brain function; without enough healthy fat and oil in your body, this thin membrane can get brittle and those electrical connections don't fire as well.

This also leads to a lack of brain function, but filling up on olive oil as well as the oil you get from peanuts and salmon and other healthy proteins nourishes the brain and keeps it functioning properly.

Chapter 4

The Basics of the Ketogenic Diet

Greatly reducing your carbohydrate intake while filling up on protein and fats is a basic way of creating your own ketogenic diet.

However, while you don't necessarily need to weigh and measure your food on this eating plan, you do want to think about just how much of each type of food you're getting. This will ensure you're reducing your carbohydrate intake enough to get your body to the ketosis stage, and will also mean you get just enough protein to be healthy without getting too many carbs from these foods.

Carbohydrate Intake

The fewer carbs you have on a ketogenic diet, the better it is for you. For most persons, you'll want to reduce your intake to less than 50 grams, and less than 20 grams is ideal.

To give you an idea of what that means, note the carbohydrate count of many common foods, grams:

- Sweet potatoes (one cup), 28
- Grapes (one cup), 28
- Banana (one medium), 27
- Chocolate milk (one cup), 26-30
- Brown rice (1/2 cup), 23.5
- Almonds (3/4 cup), 22

- Apple (one medium), 21
- Carrots (3/4 cup), 21
- Orange (one medium), 16
- Corn, peas (1/2 cup), 15
- Hot dog or hamburger bun, 15-21
- Skim milk (one cup), 12
- Oatmeal (1/2 cup), 12
- Strawberries (one cup), 11

You can see how those carbs get used up quickly, even when having a small amount of some very common foods!

To follow the ketogenic diet and reduce your carbohydrate intake, you can note the carb content of your favorite foods and create a standard meal plan for the day. You may see how you need to make adjustments in what you reduce or eliminate in order to stick within that 20-50 grams of carbs every day.

Read labels, especially of anything baked or that contains any type of flour or grains. Note the carb count of your favorite fruits in particular, since these are often high in carbohydrates.

Once you get familiar with standard carb counts, you can then usually follow a ketogenic diet without actually weighing and measuring foods for every meal.

Protein and Fat

While you want to restrict your carbohydrate intake on a ketogenic diet, you don't necessarily need to count the grams of protein you eat.

Instead, consider how your daily meals are balanced; less than 10% of what you eat should come from carbohydrates, keeping it within the 20-50 grams mentioned above. Protein should make up 15%-25% of your daily diet, and fats should comprise a good 70% of your diet.

While we'll be showing you some recipes and meal plans later in this book, consider an example of how this would work for a meal.

You might make a salad with several cups of mixed lettuces, cauliflower, peppers, onion, and cucumber. A few small chunks of tuna add to the protein count, and you use lot of olive oil and vinegar for dressing. Your carbohydrate count is then very minimal, you have a small percent of protein, and lots of healthy fats complete the meal.

Once again, thank you for reading this book, and I hope you're getting a lot of valuable information. I would greatly appreciate it if you could take 30 seconds to leave me a review for this book on Amazon.com.

Chapter 5

Safely Following the Ketogenic Diet

When you read that the ketogenic diet means filling up mostly on fats, you might wonder how this can lead to weight loss and also how it's safe. The important thing to consider is that the ketogenic diet means consuming healthy fats and proteins that are good for you, and which won't clog your arteries or have you consuming too many calories.

Let's look at this a bit more in depth.

About Fats

Dietary fats have gotten something of a bad reputation recently, as they're typically associated with actually getting fat yourself, and with clogging your arteries, causing plaque to form in your circulatory system, and increasing your risk of many heart-related diseases and health conditions.

There is some truth to these cautions, as saturated fats can be very dangerous to your health, and fats themselves are often very calorie-dense, meaning they contain a lot of calories for every gram or ounce.

Unhealthy Fats

While some cautions are in order about fats, it's good to understand the difference between saturated and unsaturated fats, and how certain fats can actually be good for you.

Saturated and unsaturated fats refer to whether or not there is a carbon bond in the chemical makeup of the fat itself; saturated fats don't have this carbon bond because they are "saturated" with hydrogen molecules.

This can seem complicated and technical, but just note that the body doesn't break down saturated fats very easily.

These are the unhealthy types that clog your arteries and cause plaque to form. They are also usually very high in calorie count, so you can be ingesting far too many calories when you have too much of these types of fats.

Saturated fats include:

- All fats made from animal products. This would include the fats in meats and dairy foods (butter, cheese, milk, yogurt).
- Palm oil.
- Palm kernel oil.
- Coconut oil.

Trans Fats

Trans fats are liquid fats that have hydrogen injected into them, to make them more solid.

This is typically done to ensure the fats are more stable during food manufacturing, or when the fats need to be shipped, such as to restaurants that use them for French fries and other dishes.

Trans fats are sometimes called "partially hydrogenated oils," referring to the hydrogen that's introduced. These fats don't break down very well in your system and can cause plaque to build up in your arteries and also raise your cholesterol.

These, too, can be considered "bad" or unhealthy fats.

Healthy Fats

Healthy fats are those that are unsaturated; these are easier for the body to break down and digest, just like other foods. These fats are actually considered healthy because the body needs fats to keep the heart and other muscles lubricated and healthy, and these fats also hydrate your organs including the eyes and skin.

Note, too, that many vitamins and trace minerals are absorbed into your body's cells by way of these healthy fats. Even if you take a multivitamin supplement, if you're not getting enough healthy fat in your system, you may still find yourself deficient of many vitamins, trace minerals, and other nutrients, simply because your body could not break them down and absorb them.

Unsaturated fats include:

- Fish oils, most specifically from salmon, tuna, mackerel, trout, and herring.
- Avocadoes.
- Nuts, especially walnuts and cashews.
- Olives and olive oil.

Protein Sources

As with fats, there are sources of protein that could be considered healthier than others, and it's good to understand this when following a ketogenic diet.

Healthy protein choices are those that don't have much saturated fat, and which aren't as calorie-dense as other choices. While following a ketogenic diet plan doesn't necessarily involve counting calories, having too many calories every day can get in the way of your weight loss and maintenance goals.

First consider the amount of fat in many sources of protein. As an example, there are different cuts of ground beef, many of which are labeled "80% lean." This means that 20% of the meat is fat!

While filling up on fats is good when following a ketogenic diet plan, beef is full of saturated or unhealthy fats that clog your arteries, so this type of protein isn't the healthiest option for you.

Note, too, that saturated fats are typically the most calorie-dense, so opting for protein with saturated fats will mean taking in more calories than you may need.

In turn, you may not lose as much weight when following the ketogenic diet as you expect. Filling up on lean protein choices, or those with unsaturated fat and which aren't as calorie dense, is the better option.

Consider some lean sources of protein that have lower amounts of saturated fat, or none at all, and which are better choices when following a ketogenic diet plan:

- Fish of any sort, but especially tuna, mackerel, and salmon.
- White meat poultry, including chicken and turkey. Dark meat has a bit more fat than the white meat, but not usually as much as beef.
- Eggs are very low in fat and high in protein.
- Skim milk and dairy products made from skim milk, including low-fat cheese and yogurt.
- Beans of all sorts, and foods made from beans and legumes including hummus.
- Soy.
- Nuts, especially walnuts.

One reason that some people who follow a ketogenic diet don't get the results they want when it comes to weight loss and reducing their cholesterol is that they fill up on unhealthy choices for fat and protein, not considering if they're ingesting lots of calorie-dense, saturated fat.

Instead, if you make these lean protein choices the main staple of your diet and opt for unsaturated, healthy fats, you'll see better and faster results with weight loss and won't risk high cholesterol levels.

Enjoying this book?

Check out my other best sellers!

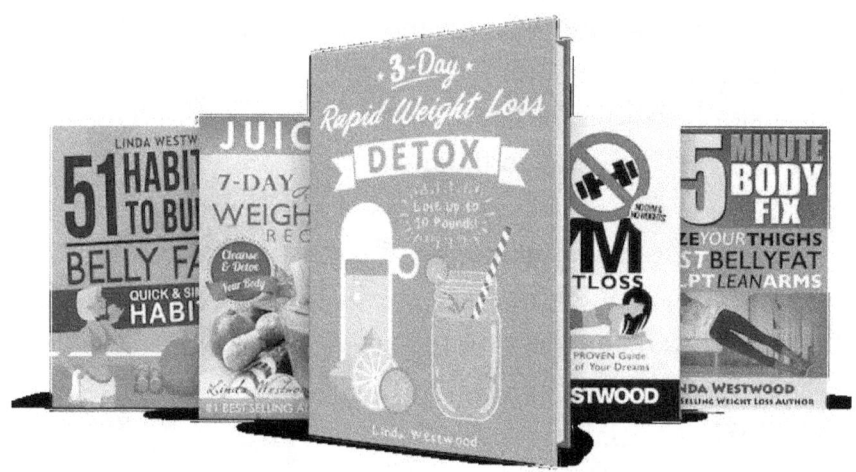

Get your next book on sale here:

TopFitnessAdvice.com/go/books

Ketogenic Meal Plan Recipes

To get started on the ketogenic diet, check out some great recipes that you can try right from your own kitchen!

One note to remember; some of these recipes may include ingredients you've never tried before, such as stevia sweetener or xanthan gum.

Chances are, these ingredients can easily be found in the baking aisle at your local grocery store, but you may have just passed them by since you've never used them before!

These items can also be found online at sites such as Amazon.com and those that sell commercial cooking supplies.

These ingredients may sound a bit unfamiliar to you, but rest assured they're very natural and are often used in commercial kitchens to prepare certain dishes that are low-cal or low-carb.

Once you get started using them, you may wonder how you ever cooked without them!

So if you're ready to get started with the ketogenic diet, let's get going!

Pumpkin Waffles

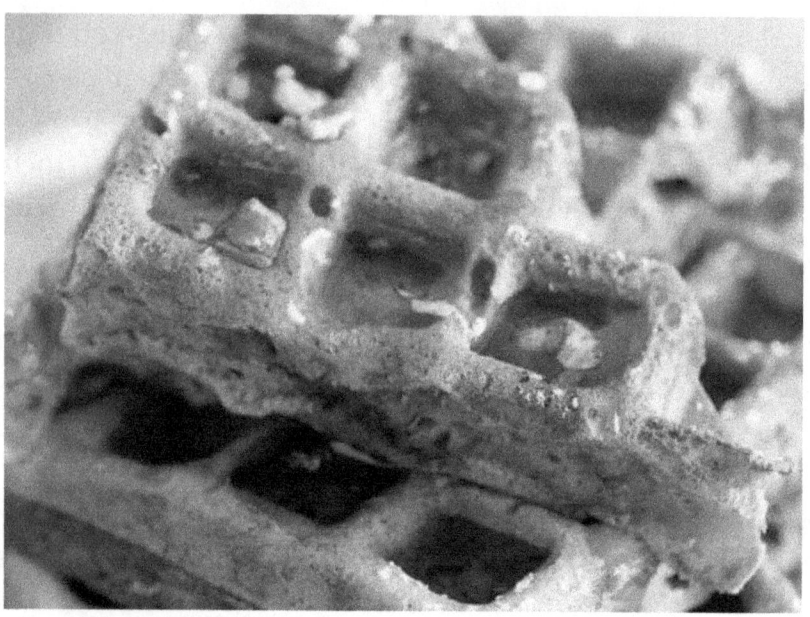

Ingredients

- 1/2 cup almond flour
- 2 tbsp. flaxseed meal
- 1/3 cup coconut milk
- 1/4 cup canned pumpkin
- 1-1/2 tsp. pumpkin pie spice
- 1 tsp. vanilla extract
- 1 tsp. baking powder
- 2 large Eggs
- 3 tbsp. artificial sweetener
- 7 drops stevia

Directions

1. Mix the wet ingredients together in a bowl. Gently sift in the dry ingredients and fold the batter.

2. Use coconut oil cooking spray to grease your waffle iron. Cook until the waffles are golden brown. Serve with just a sprinkling of cinnamon.

Makes 2 servings.

Cauliflower Waffles

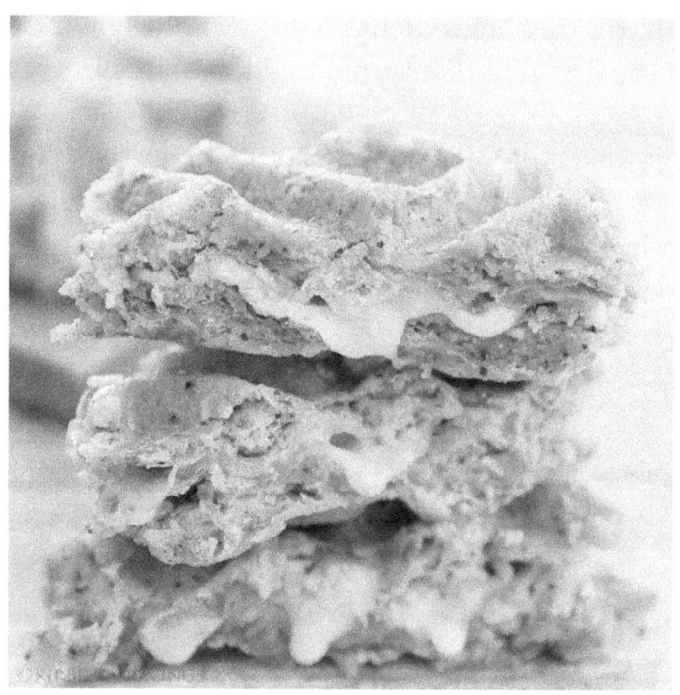

Ingredients

- 1-1/2 cup cauliflower
- 1/2 cup mozzarella cheese
- 1/4 cup parmesan cheese
- 1/2 cup cheddar cheese
- 3 eggs
- 3 tbsp. chives
- 1/2 tsp. onion powder
- 1/2 tsp. garlic powder
- 1/4 tsp. red pepper flakes

Directions

1. Grate the cauliflower and cheeses together using a food processor. Add the eggs, chives, and seasoning (adjust amounts of seasoning to taste; add a pinch of salt and pepper as well, if preferred).

2. Cook in waffle maker about 8 minutes on one side, then flip and cook another 8 minutes on other side, or until golden brown.

Makes 4 servings.

Others who are considering purchasing this book would love to know what you think. If you could spare a few seconds, they would greatly appreciate reading an honest review from you. Simply visit the page on Amazon.com.

Cheese and Veggie Frittata

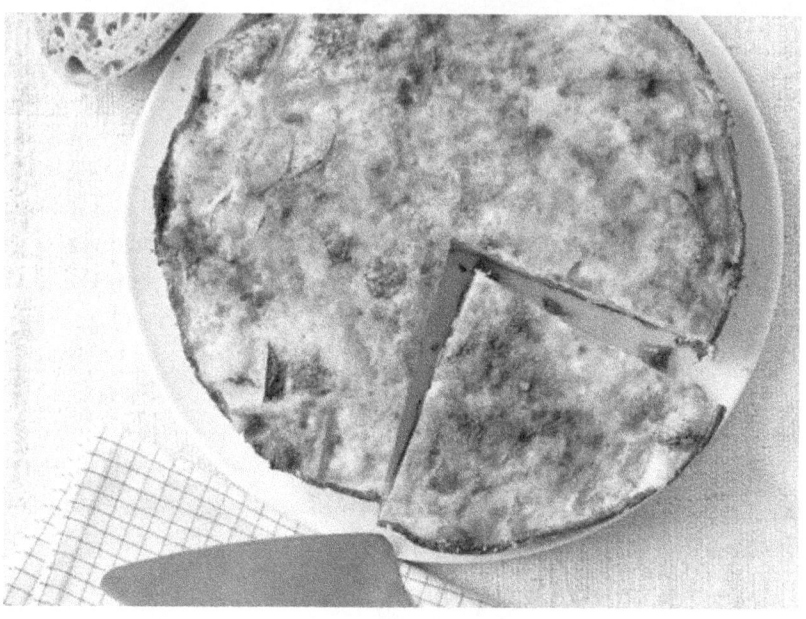

Ingredients

- 7 slices bacon
- 1 tbsp. olive oil
- 1 medium red bell pepper, diced
- 4 large mushroom caps, sliced
- 8 eggs
- 1/4 cup heavy cream
- 1/4 cup grated parmesan cheese
- 1/2 cup fresh basil, chopped
- 4 oz. mozzarella cheese, cut into cubes
- 2 oz. grated goat cheese

Directions

1. Preheat oven to 350F. Add olive oil to an oven-safe frying pan and cook bacon until crisp, then remove from pan and chop; return to pan. Add bell pepper and cook until soft.

2. Add mushroom caps and stir well, and allow mushrooms to absorb the oil in the pan. Meanwhile, in separate bowl, mix eggs, cream, and parmesan cheese together. Once combined, use whisk to mix thoroughly.

3. Add basil to the top of the bacon mixture and let it wilt. Then, spread mozzarella cheese cubes on top.

4. Pour egg mixture into the pan but combine ingredients by lifting the bacon mixture, not stirring; this allows the egg mixture to reach the bottom of the pan.

5. Remove pan from heat, add goat cheese to the top, and bake for 6-8 minutes. Move pan to oven broiler and broil for another 4 minutes.

6. Remove the frittata from the pan by flipping it onto parchment paper or a serving plate. Slice with pizza cutter.

Makes 6 servings.

Bacon Avocado Muffins

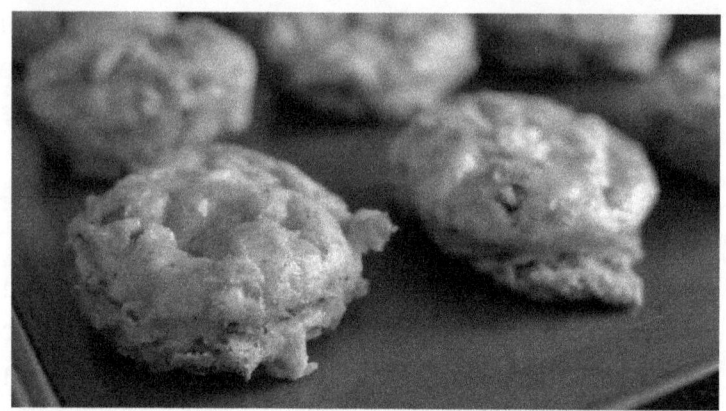

Ingredients

- 5 eggs
- 1/2 cup Almond Flour
- 1/4 cup Flaxseed Meal
- 1-1/2 tbsp. Psyllium Husk Powder
- 1 tsp. Minced Garlic
- 1 tsp. Dried Cilantro
- 1 tsp. Dried Chives
- 1/4 tsp. Red Chili Flakes
- 1-1/2 cup Coconut Milk
- 1-1/2 tbsp. Lemon Juice
- 5 Slices Bacon
- 2 tbsp. Butter
- 2 medium Avocados
- 4-1/2 oz. Colby Jack Cheese
- 3 medium Spring Onions
- 1 tsp. Baking Powder

Directions

1. In a bowl, mix together eggs, almond flour, flax, psyllium, spices, coconut milk and lemon juice. Set aside and cook the bacon. Just before the bacon is crisp, add the butter.

2. Dice the avocado insides, the cheese, and the onions, and mix with the baking powder. Remove bacon from pan, dice, and add to avocado mixture. Fold this into egg mixture. Bake in ungreased muffin tins at 350F for 25 minutes.

Makes 12 muffins.

Crock-pot Chicken Soup

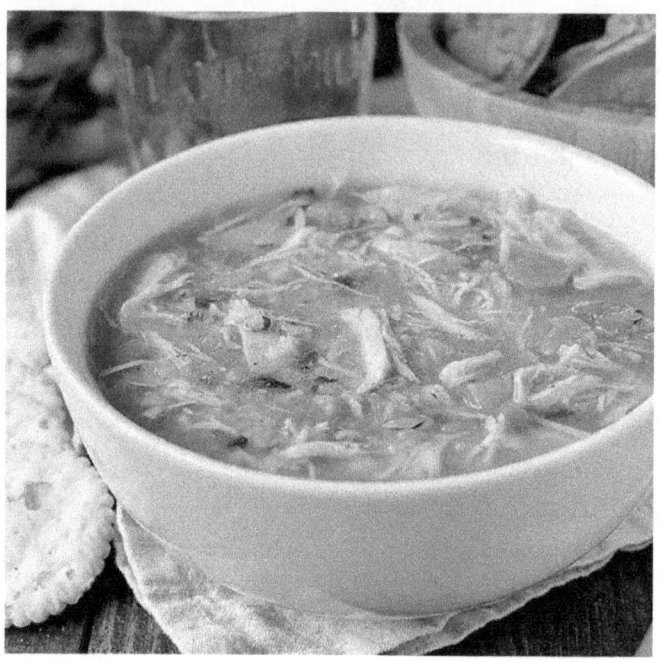

Ingredients

- 1-1/2 pounds Chicken Thighs, deboned and chunked
- 1 tsp. Onion Powder
- 1 tsp. Garlic Powder
- 1/2 tsp. Celery Seed
- 1/4 cup Butter
- 1/3 cup Hot Sauce
- 3 cups Beef Broth
- 1 cup Heavy Cream
- 2 oz. Cream Cheese
- 1/4 tsp. Xanthan Gum

Directions

1. Add chicken to crock-pot. Add remaining ingredients except for cream, cream cheese, and xanthan gum. Set crock-pot to low and let cook for 6 hours.

2. Next, remove the chicken and shred with a fork; set aside. Add remaining three ingredients to crock-pot and mix well.

3. Add chicken back to mixture and stir again. Let sit in crock-pot until reheated; serve.

Makes 5 servings.

Grilled Cheese

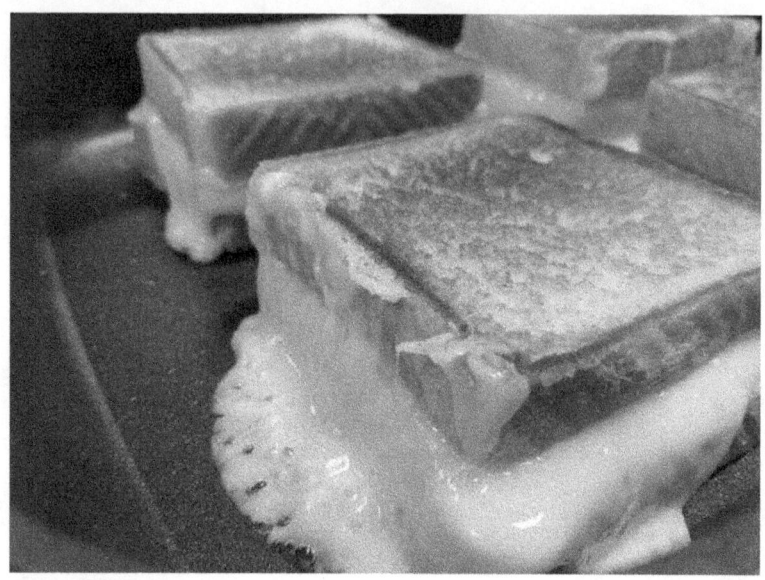

Ingredients

- 2 tbsp. Soft Butter (plus one pat for grilling)
- 2 tbsp. Almond Flour
- 1-1/2 tbsp. Psyllium Husk Powder
- 1/2 tsp. Baking Powder
- 2 large Eggs
- 2 oz cheddar cheese

Directions

1. Add all the ingredients except the eggs and cheese in a square, microwave-safe bowl and mix together thoroughly, until a soft dough is formed.

2. Add the two eggs and continue to blend until the dough is mixed and thick. Let this sit in the bottom of the bowl and push down with a spoon or spatula so the top is as flat as possible.

3. Microwave for 90 seconds to two minutes, until the batter is cooked into bread. Turn the bowl upside down to remove the bread, then slice it horizontally, for two flat pieces.

4. Heat the pat of butter in a frying pan and set down one slice of bread; add the cheddar cheese over this and cover with second slice. Grill as desired.

Makes 1 sandwich.

Enchilada Soup

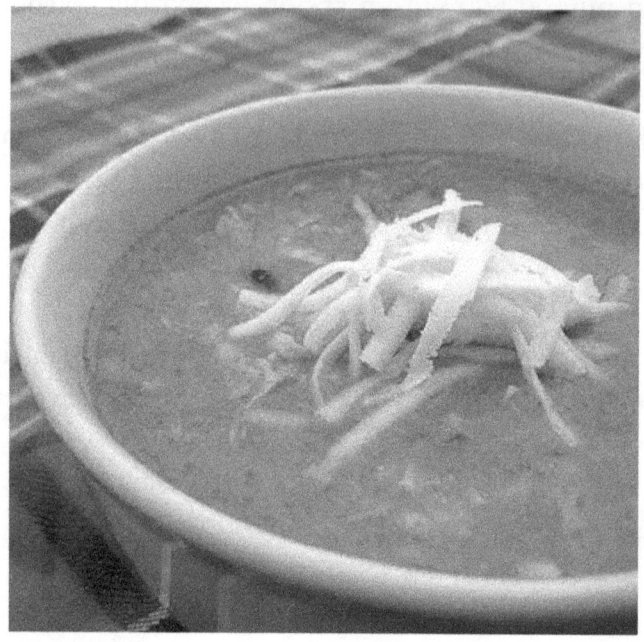

Ingredients

- 3 tbsp. Olive Oil
- 3 stalks Celery, diced
- 1 medium Red Bell Pepper, diced
- 2 tsp. Garlic, minced
- 1 cup Diced Fresh Tomatoes
- 2 tsp. Cumin
- 1 tsp. Oregano
- 1 tsp. Chili Powder
- 1/2 tsp. Cayenne Pepper
- 1/2 cup Cilantro, chopped
- 4 cups Chicken Broth
- 8 oz. Cream Cheese

- 6 oz. Chicken, shredded
- 1/2 Medium Lime, juiced

Directions

1. In a large pot, heat the olive oil over high heat. Add the celery, bell pepper, and garlic. Let this cook until vegetables are tender. Add tomatoes and spices, stir, then add chicken broth and stir again.

2. Bring to a boil, stir in cream cheese, continue stirring to mix, and then reduce the heat and let simmer for 20 minutes.

3. Once simmered, add the chicken and squeeze the lime juice over the top of the pan. Let heat to desired temperature and serve.

Makes 4 servings.

Ginger Glaze for Salmon

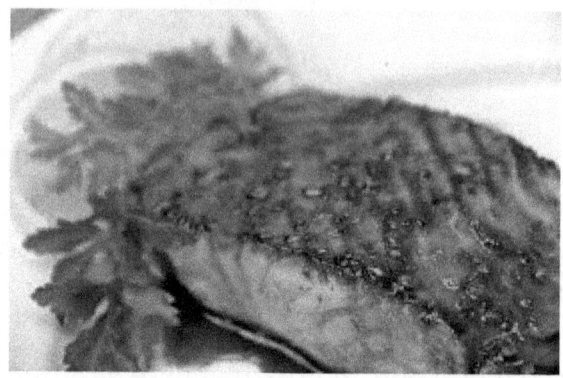

This glaze will cover about 10 ounces of salmon (approximately 2 fillets), or any other thick fish you might have with ginger.

Ingredients

- 2 tbsp. Soy Sauce
- 1 tbsp. Rice Vinegar
- 1 tsp. Minced Ginger
- 2 tsp. Minced Garlic
- 2 tsp. Sesame Oil
- 1 tbsp. Sugar Free Ketchup
- 2 tbsp. White Wine

Directions

1. Mix first 4 ingredients in a flat container or dish; once mixed, add in fish and allow to marinate for about 15 minutes.

2. Use the sesame oil in a warm pan and heat until slightly smoking; add fish and cook until crispy, then flip.

3. Add the marinade liquid to the pan and allow to boil and cover the fish. Remove fish from pan and add ketchup and wine to marinade. Let simmer to reduce and then drizzle over the fish.

Makes 2 servings.

Stuffed Avocados

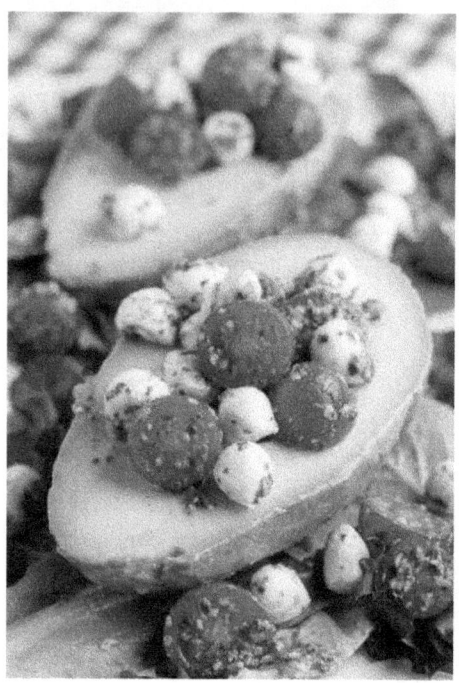

Ingredients

- 6 large Hard Boiled Eggs, chopped
- 1/3 medium Red Onion, chopped
- 3 stalks Celery, chopped
- 4 tbsp. Mayonnaise
- 2 tsp. Brown Mustard
- 2 tbsp. Fresh Lime Juice
- 1 tsp. Hot Sauce
- 1/2 tsp. Cumin
- 3 medium Avocados

Directions

1. In a bowl, mix all ingredients except avocados. Stir gently so chopped egg pieces don't get crushed.

2. Slice avocados horizontally and remove the pit. Add a scoop of egg mixture to this "well" or hollowed area. Serve chilled.

Makes 6 servings.

Chicken in Zucchini

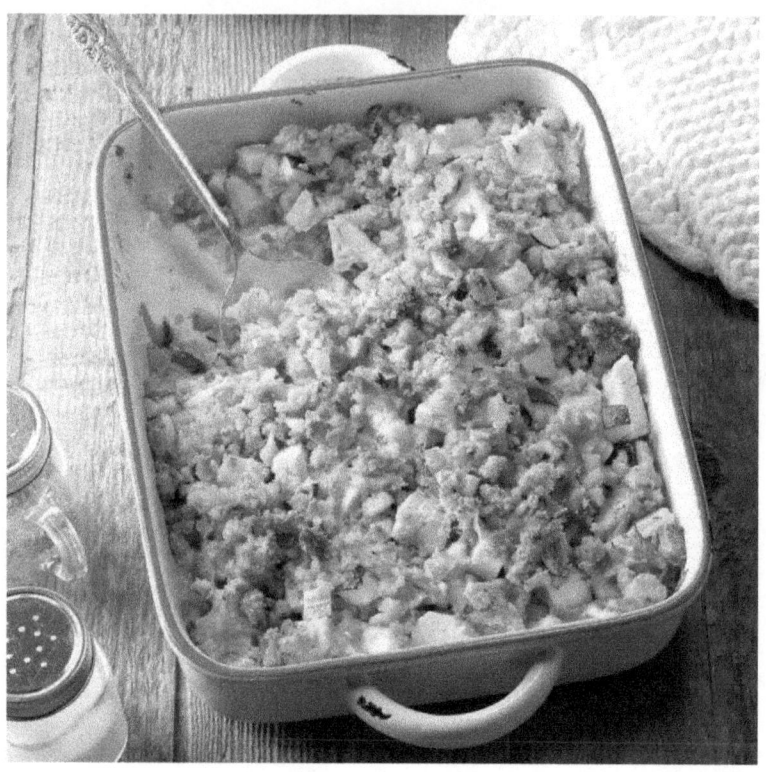

Ingredients

- 2 large zucchini, cut horizontally, slightly hollowed out
- 2 tbsp. Butter, melted
- 1 cup Broccoli, diced
- 6 oz. Cooked Chicken, shredded (rotisserie chicken leftovers work well)
- 2 tbsp. Sour Cream
- 3 oz. Cheddar Cheese, shredded
- 1 stalk Green Onion

Directions

1. Preheat oven to 400F. Pour the butter evenly over the inside of the zucchini halves, place them on a cookie sheet, and put them in the oven. Allow them to cook for 20 minutes while you prepare the filling.

2. In large mixing bowl, mix the broccoli, chicken, and sour cream. Remove zucchini from oven and fill with chicken mixture.

3. Sprinkle cheddar cheese over the top and return the zucchini to the oven, allowing them to cook another 5 minutes or until the cheese is melted.

Makes 2 servings.

Pumpkin Muffins

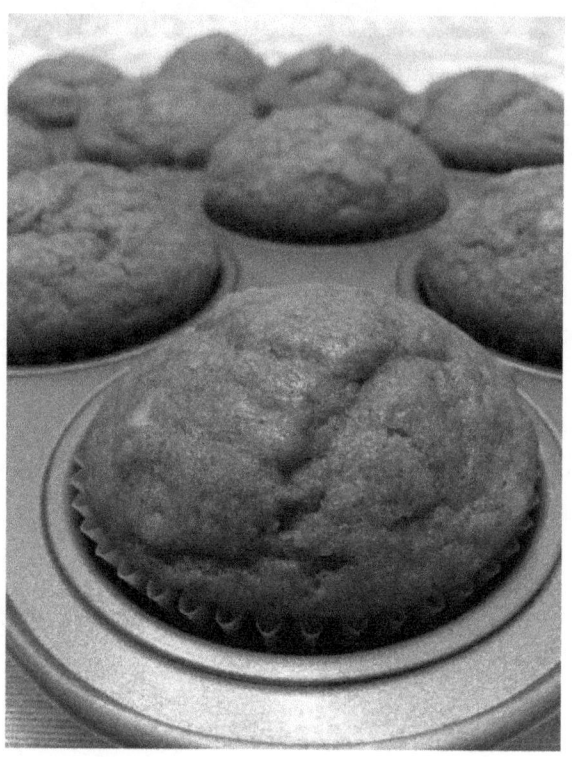

Ingredients

- 3/4 cup canned pumpkin
- 1/4 cup sugarless sunflower butter
- 1 large egg
- 1/2 cup erythritol sweetener
- 1/4 cup coconut flour, sifted
- 2 tbsp. flaxseed
- 1 tsp. cinnamon
- 1/2 tsp. nutmeg
- 1/2 tsp. baking soda

- 1/2 tsp. baking powder
- 1/4 tsp. salt

Directions

1. Preheat oven to 350F and lightly grease muffin tins. In large mixing bowl, mix pumpkin, butter, and egg.

2. Gently fold in dry ingredients and mix. Spoon into muffin tins and bake 15 minutes.

Makes 16 muffins.

Pizza Casserole

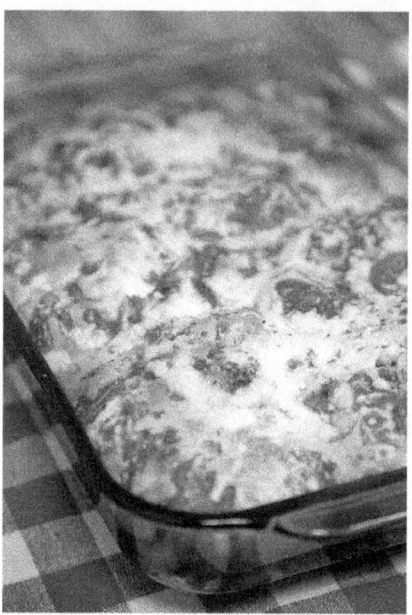

Ingredients

- 1 medium head cauliflower, diced
- 1 tbsp. butter
- 1 small yellow onion, diced
- 1 clove garlic, crushed
- 2 tbsp. balsamic vinegar
- 1 cup heavy cream
- 6 oz. cream cheese, chunked
- 3 tbsp. tomato paste
- 3 cups mozzarella cheese, divided
- 1/2 tsp. dried oregano
- 1 tbsp. fresh basil
- 1 tsp. sea salt

- 1/4 tsp. freshly ground pepper
- 3 oz. package thinly sliced pepperoni

Directions

1. Preheat oven to 350F. Steam cauliflower until crisp but tender. Set aside.

2. In large skillet, melt butter. Add onion and cook until tender. Add garlic and cook for one minute. Add vinegar and continue cooking until mixture thickens.

3. Add cream, cream cheese, and tomato paste and stir, then stir in 1 cup of the mozzarella cheese. Simmer until thickened. Add seasonings and stir.

4. In 9-inch pan, spread half of the cauliflower and then arrange pepperoni slices on top. Add one cup of the remaining mozzarella cheese. Add remaining cauliflower and then pepperoni, and then add the cream sauce. Add the remaining mozzarella cheese on top.

5. Bake for 20 to 30 minutes until bubbly, and allow to cool slightly before serving.

Makes 9 servings.

I hope you have learned something from this book so far and would greatly appreciate it if you could leave an honest review on Amazon.com.

Raspberry Popsicles

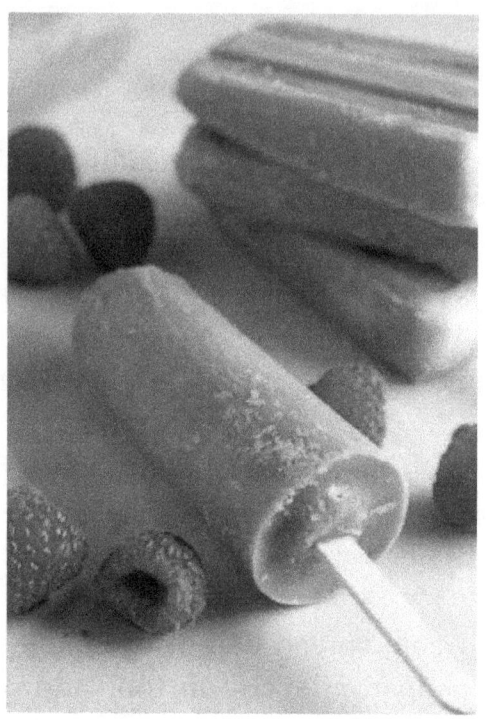

Ingredients

- 100g Raspberries
- Juice of 1/2 Lemon
- 1/4 cup Coconut Oil
- 1 cup Coconut Milk
- 1/4 cup Sour Cream
- 1/4 cup Heavy Cream
- 1/2 tsp. Guar Gum
- 20 drops stevia sweetener

Directions

1. Blend all ingredients in a food processor or juicer until completely blended. Strain through a sieve to remove all raspberry seeds and pulp left behind.

2. Pour the mixture into popsicle molds, add sticks, and freeze for at least 2 hours or overnight before serving.

Makes 6 popsicles.

Asian Salad

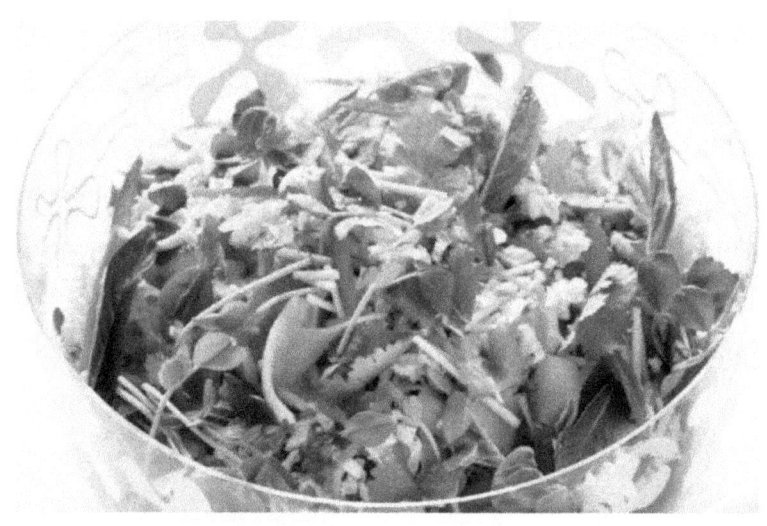

Ingredients

- 12 oz. bag broccoli slaw
- 2 tbsp. coconut oil
- 1 tbsp. coconut amino or nectar
- 1 tsp. fresh ginger, grated
- 1/2 tsp. salt
- 1/4 tsp. pepper
- 1/2 cup full fat plain yogurt
- 1/2 tbsp. sesame seeds

Directions

1. Cook broccoli slaw in coconut oil in large skillet, covered, for 7 minutes. Add coconut amino or nectar, ginger, and salt and pepper if desired.

2. Remove from heat, add yogurt and sesame seeds, and stir. Serve while still warm.

Serves 8.

Pumpkin Bars

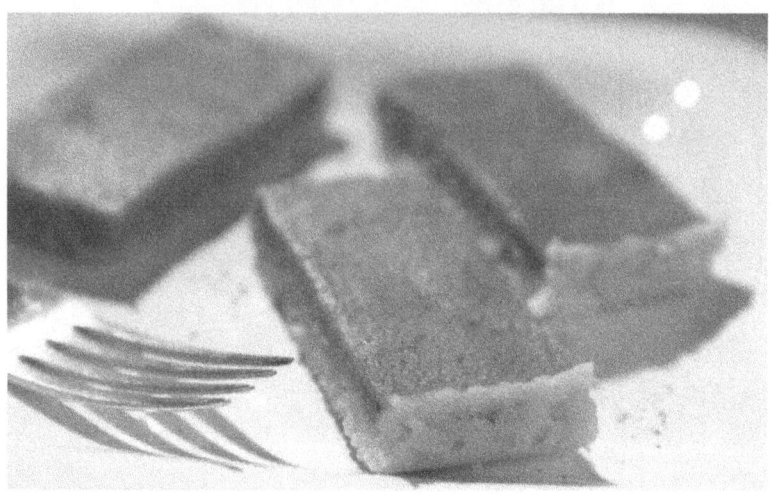

Ingredients

- 1 cup coconut flour, sifted
- 1/2 cup erythritol
- 1 tbsp. unsweetened baking cocoa powder
- 1-1/4 tsp. ground ginger
- 1 tsp. ground cinnamon
- 1/2 tsp. baking soda
- 1/2 tsp. salt
- 1/4 tsp. ground nutmeg
- 1/2 cup coconut oil
- 2 large eggs
- 2 tsp. pure vanilla extract
- 8-ounce cream cheese, softened at room temperature
- 1/2 cup pure pumpkin puree
- 1 large egg
- 1/4 cup erythritol

- 1/2 tsp. ground cinnamon
- 1/4 tsp. ground ginger
- Pinch of ground nutmeg

Directions

1. Preheat oven to 350F. Whisk together first 8 ingredients. Once mixed, add coconut oil, eggs, and vanilla and mix completely. Set aside 1 cup of this mixture; add remaining mixture to 8x8 greased baking pan. Press down firmly and then set aside.

2. In separate bowl, mix remaining ingredients until creamed together thoroughly and spread over base mixture in pan. Add remaining 1 cup of mixture to top and spread evenly.

3. Bake 25-30 minutes and then allow to cool for 2 hours in refrigerator before serving.

Makes 16 servings.

Cheese Waffles

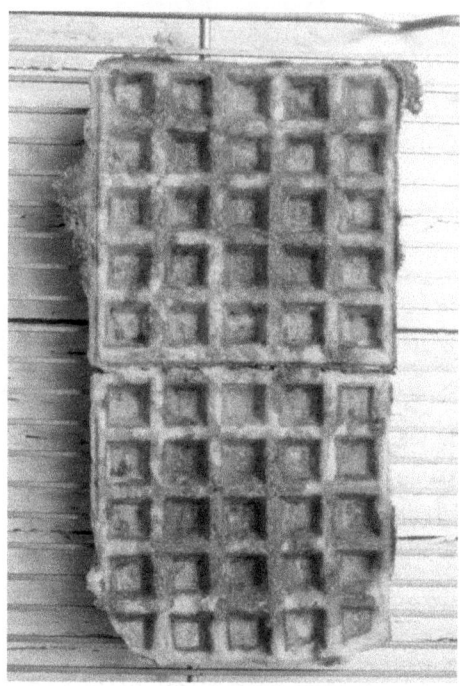

Ingredients

- 1-1/3 cup coconut flour, sifted
- 3 tsp. baking powder
- 1 tsp. dried ground sage
- 1/2 tsp. salt
- 1/4 tsp. garlic powder
- 2 cups canned coconut milk
- 1/2 cup water
- 2 whole eggs
- 3 tbsp. coconut oil, melted
- 1 cup cheddar cheese, shredded

Directions

1. In large bowl, whisk together flour, baking powder, sage, salt, and garlic powder. Add liquid ingredients and stir until batter is runny.

2. Mix in cheddar cheese. Cook in waffle iron according to desired doneness and cut into 12 servings when finished.

Makes 12 small waffles.

Skillet Bacon and Eggs

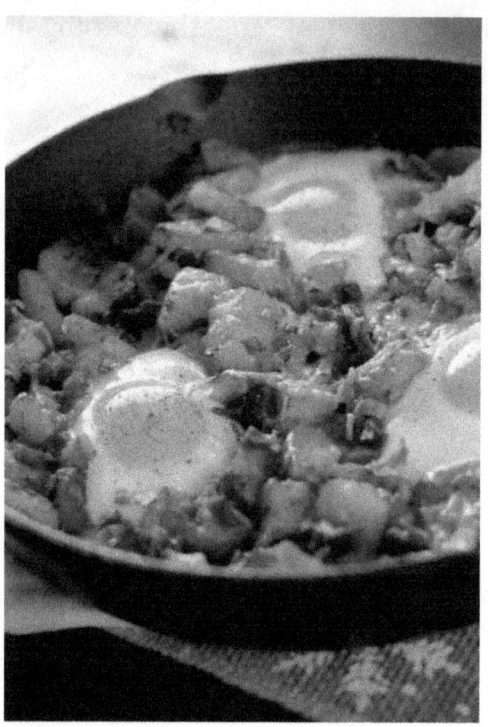

Ingredients

- 1 tbsp. butter
- 8 slices meaty bacon
- 1 carrot, peeled into thin strips
- 1/2 cup chopped broccoli or cauliflower
- 1/2 cup finely chopped celery
- 1/2 large white onion, peeled and chopped into small pieces
- 4 large organic eggs
- 1/2 cup shredded Colby Jack cheese

Directions

1. Melt butter in skillet and add bacon and vegetables. Sauté for about 20 minutes, until bacon is crisp and vegetables are cooked through. Spread this mixture evenly over the pan and then make four "wells" in the mixture, for the eggs.

2. Add eggs to each of these wells and cook, covered, until the eggs are cooked through according to your preference. Sprinkle cheese over the top, remove the pan from the heat and cover for 2 or 3 more minutes to melt the cheese and then serve.

Serves 4.

Strawberry Protein Shake

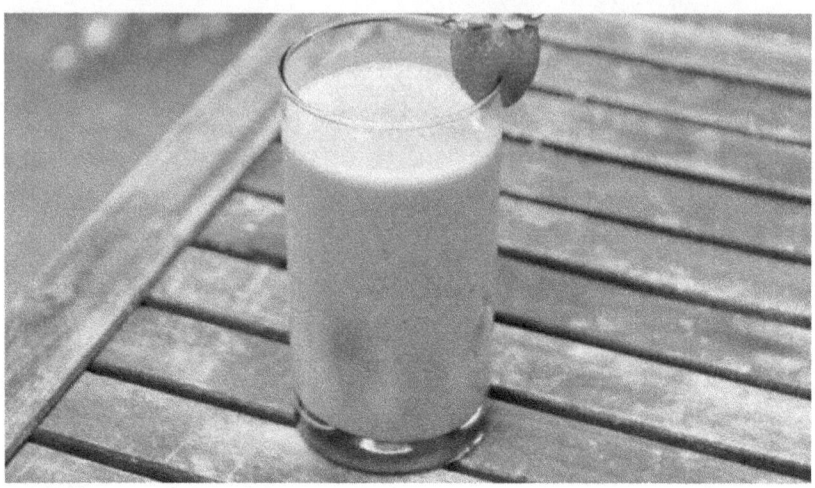

Ingredients

- 16 ounces unsweetened almond milk
- 4-ounce heavy cream
- 2 scoops Chocolate Whey Isolate powder, any variety
- 1 tbsp. Sugar Free Strawberry Syrup
- 1/2 cup crushed ice

Directions

1. Put all ingredients in blender. Blend until smooth.

Makes 2 servings.

Orange Coconut Shake

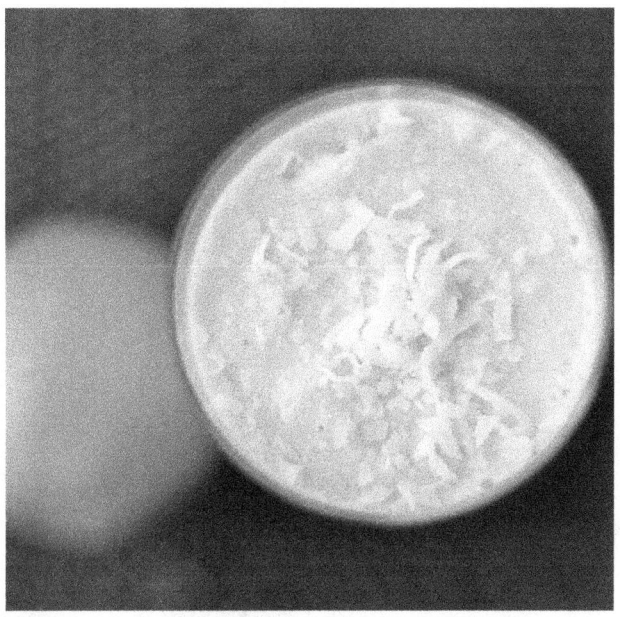

Ingredients

- 16 ounces unsweetened almond milk
- 4-ounce heavy cream
- 2 scoops Whey Protein Powder, any variety
- 1 tablespoon of sugar free Coconut Syrup
- 1/2 cup crushed ice

Directions

1. Put all ingredients in blender. Blend until smooth.

Makes 2 servings.

White Chocolate Protein Shake

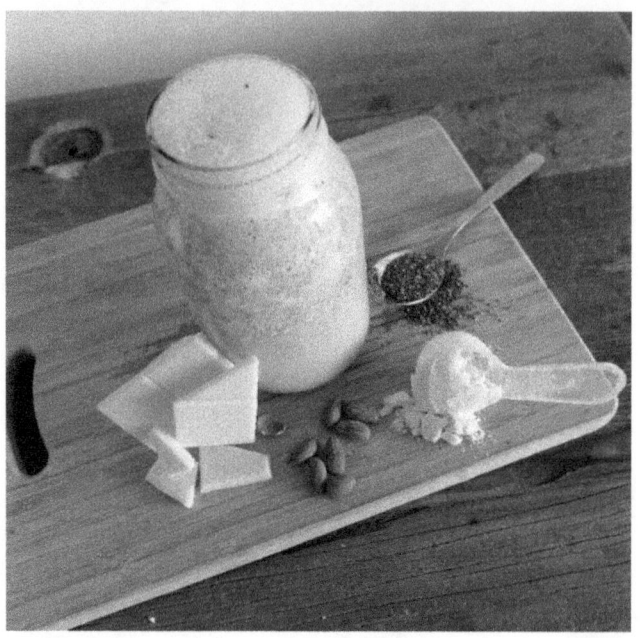

Ingredients

- 16 ounces unsweetened almond milk
- 4-ounce heavy cream
- 2 scoops Vanilla Whey Powder, any variety
- 1 tablespoon Sugar Free White Chocolate syrup
- 1/2 cup crushed ice

Directions

1. Put all ingredients in blender. Blend until smooth.

Makes 2 servings.

Chocolate Protein Shake

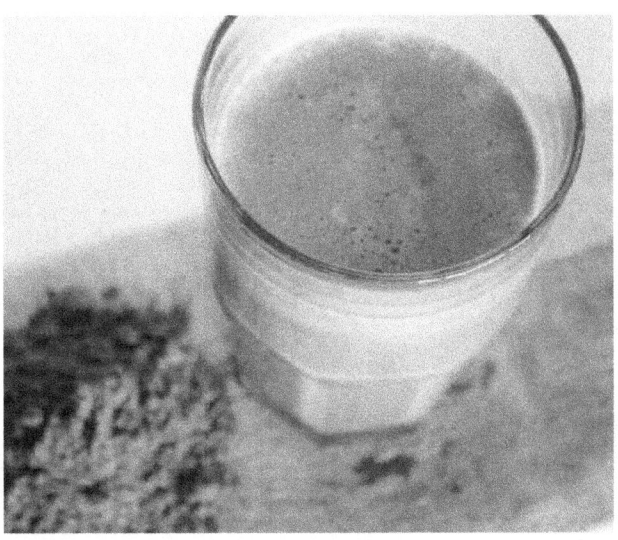

Ingredients

- 12 ounces unsweetened almond milk
- ounce heavy cream
- 1/2 cup frozen strawberries
- 1 scoop Chocolate Whey Powder, any variety
- 2-3 drops of vanilla flavored stevia
- 1 tbsp. unsweetened cocoa powder
- 1 tbsp. gelatin powder

Directions

1. Put all ingredients in blender. Blend until smooth.

Makes 1 serving.

Peanut Butter Protein Shake

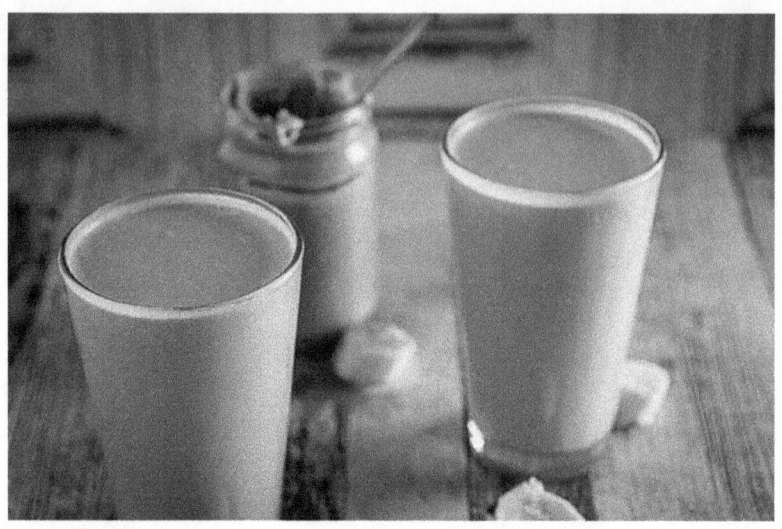

Ingredients

- 1 cup unsweetened almond milk
- 1 scoop whey protein powder, either chocolate or vanilla
- 1 tsp. flaxseed
- 1 tsp. peanut butter
- 1 tbsp. unsweetened cocoa powder
- Crushed ice

Directions

1. Put all ingredients into a blender. Blend until smooth.

Makes 1 protein shake.

Meatloaf

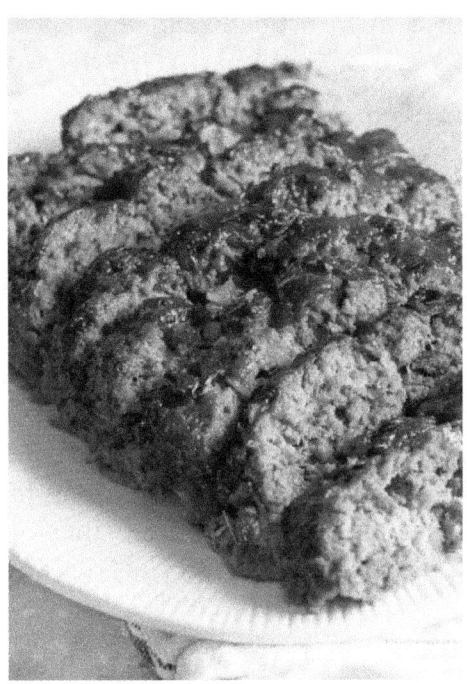

Ingredients

- 1/2 cup almond flour
- 1/2 cup dry grated Parmesan cheese
- 2 tbsp. butter for sautéing
- 1 chopped white onion
- 5 garlic cloves, minced
- 1 cup chopped green pepper
- 2 large eggs
- 1 tbsp. fresh basil leaves, chopped
- 1 tbsp. thyme leaves
- 1/4 cup minced parsley leaves
- 1 tsp. salt

- 1/2 tsp. ground black pepper
- 2 tsp. Dijon mustard
- 2 tbsp. Low Carb Barbecue sauce
- 1/4 cup heavy cream
- 1/2 tsp. unflavored gelatin
- 2 pounds ground beef
- 1 pound Italian sausage

Directions

1. Preheat oven to 350F and grease 10x15 baking pan.

2. In large mixing bowl, whisk flour and parmesan cheese together. Set aside. Heat butter in skillet; add onion, garlic, and pepper, and sauté until softened. Set aside.

3. In second bowl, whisk eggs with spices, salt, pepper, mustard, sauce, and cream. Add gelatin and let stand 5 minutes or until firm. Add onion mixture and mix well; set aside.

4. On large cutting board, mix beef and sausage together. Place in large mixing bowl; add eggs mixture and mix well. Add flour mixture and mix evenly.

5. Place in baking dish, forming into loaf; flatten on top so mixture cooks evenly. Bake until brown, about 1 hour. Cool for 20 minutes before slicing and serving.

Makes 12 servings.

Taco Meatballs

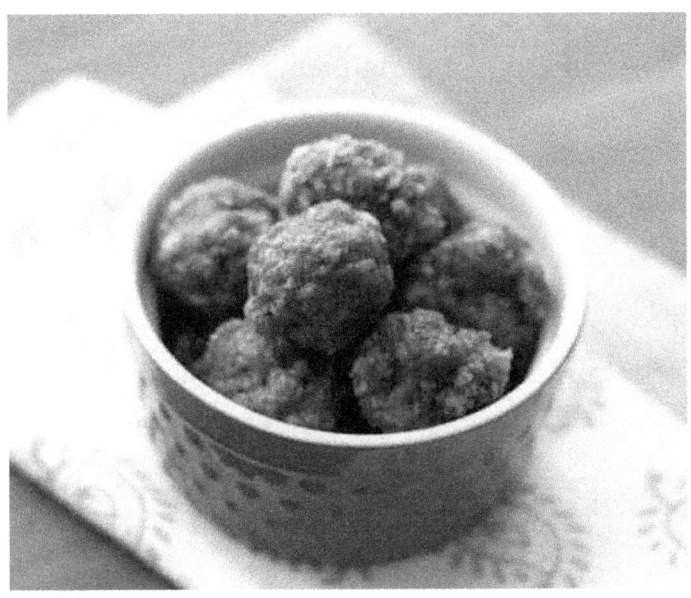

Ingredients

- 4-ounce white onion, minced
- 1 tbsp. butter
- 1 cup cold ricotta cheese
- 1 egg
- 1-1/2 tsp. minced garlic
- 1-1/2 tsp. sea salt
- 1/2 tsp. freshly black pepper
- 1-1/2 tsp. ground cumin
- 1-1/2 tsp. chili powder
- 1 tsp. ground coriander
- 4 ounces Colby Jack cheese, shredded
- 1 pound ground beef

Directions

1. Preheat oven to 350F. Sauté onions in butter until cooked through and then remove from heat.

2. Meanwhile, combine ricotta cheese and egg; whisk until smooth. Add spices along with a pinch of salt and pepper if preferred, and mix well.

3. Add onions and Colby jack cheese; mix. Add beef; mix. Form into meatballs, place on cookie sheet, and bake in preheated oven about 20 minutes.

Makes about 25 meatballs.

Mexican Layer Bowl

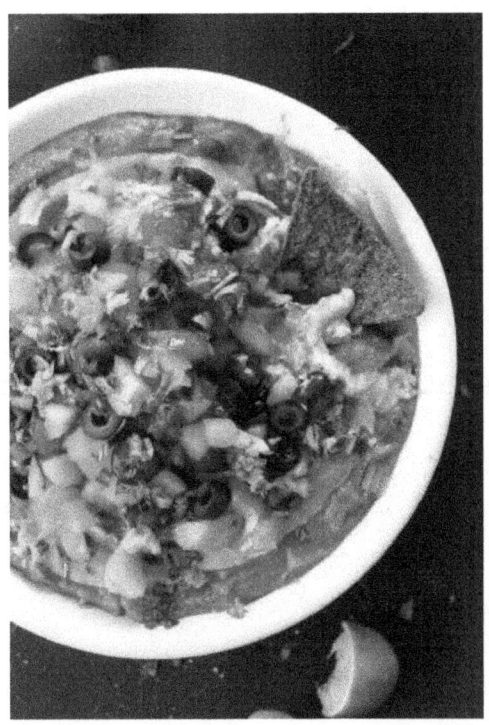

Ingredients

- 2 ripe avocados, cut into chunks
- 1 tbsp. lime juice
- 1/4 cup fresh cilantro, chopped
- 1/4 cup white onion, chopped
- 1 small tomato, seeded and chopped
- 1 tsp. minced garlic
- 1/2 tsp. sea salt
- 2 pounds ground beef
- 1/2 cup water
- 1/4 cup taco seasoning

- 2 cups sour cream
- 2 cups shredded lettuce
- 2 cups shredded cheddar cheese

Directions

1. In mixing bowl, mash together first 7 ingredients; cover and refrigerate while you complete the next steps.

2. In medium skillet, cook ground beef until cooked through. Add water and taco seasoning and stir. Reduce heat and simmer for 10 minutes.

3. Transfer this to four individual bowls and then top with sour cream, the guacamole mixture above, lettuce, and then cheddar cheese.

Makes 4 servings.

Low Carb Basil Pesto

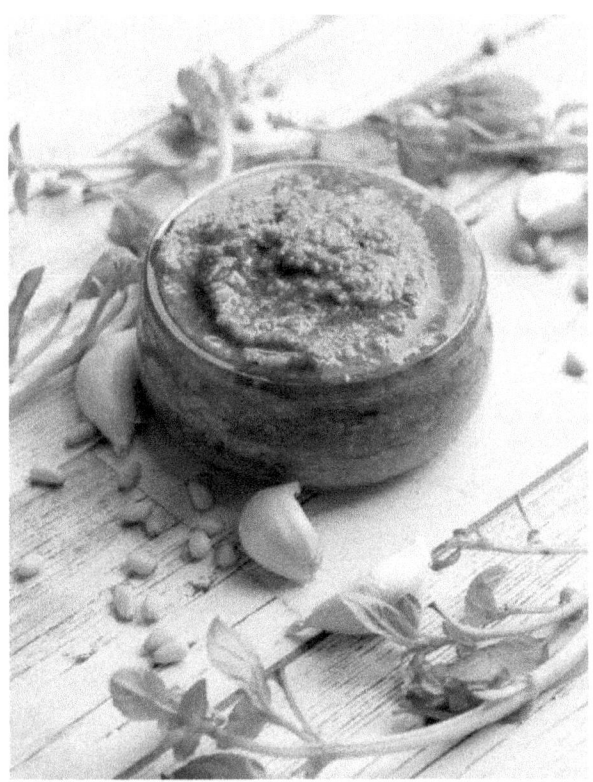

Ingredients

- 3 cups fresh basil
- 1/3 cup plus 2 tbsp. extra virgin olive oil
- 1/3 cup fresh pine nuts
- 2 garlic cloves
- 1/2 cup grated parmesan cheese
- kosher salt and pepper, to taste

Directions

1. Add all ingredients except the 2 tablespoons olive oil to food processor or blender. Process on low as you gradually add in the remaining olive oil.

2. Stop and scrap the sides repeatedly throughout the process until ingredients are smooth.

Makes about 2 cups pesto.

Potato-Not-Potato Salad

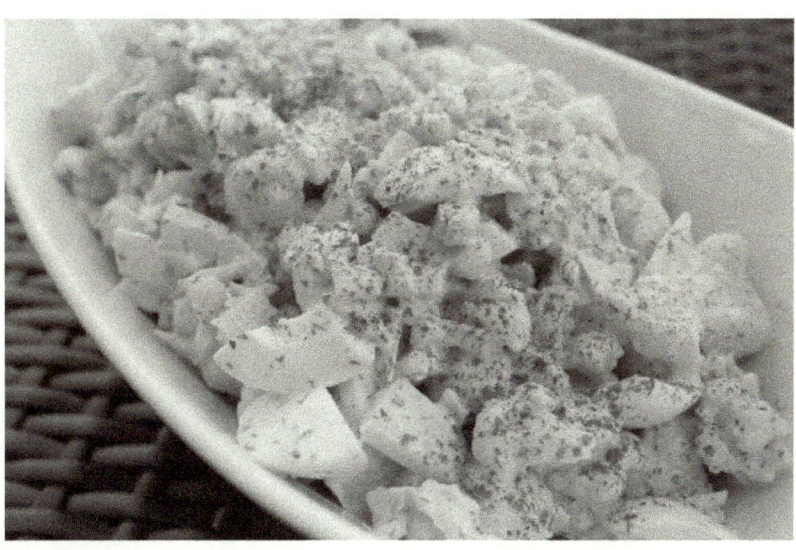

Ingredients

- 1 head cauliflower, cut into chunks
- 2 stalks celery, diced
- 1 small onion, finely chopped
- 1 tbsp. parsley, chopped
- 2 large eggs, hard boiled, peeled, and diced
- 2 tbsp. low-carb mayo
- 1 tbsp. Dijon mustard
- 1/2 tsp. sea salt

Directions

1. Chop cauliflower until diced; steam in large pan until tender. Drain and place in large bowl to cool.

2. Once cooled, add celery, onion, parsley, and egg. Gently stir in mayonnaise, mustard, and salt. Place in refrigerator for several minutes to chill and allow to set.

Makes 4 servings.

Easiest Cucumber Salad

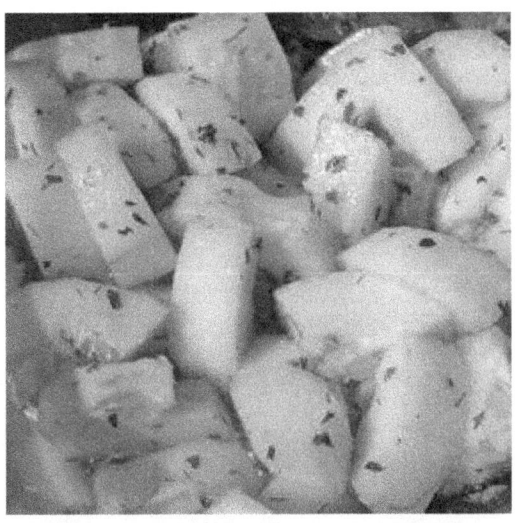

Ingredients

- 2 large cucumbers, peeled
- 1/2 cup apple cider vinegar
- 1/2 teaspoon coarse sea salt

Directions

1. Slice cucumber and then cut slices into quarters. Place in medium glass bowl and cover with vinegar, then sprinkle with salt.

2. Refrigerate for several minutes so cucumbers can absorb mixture, then serve.

Makes 4 servings.

Chicken Olive Casserole

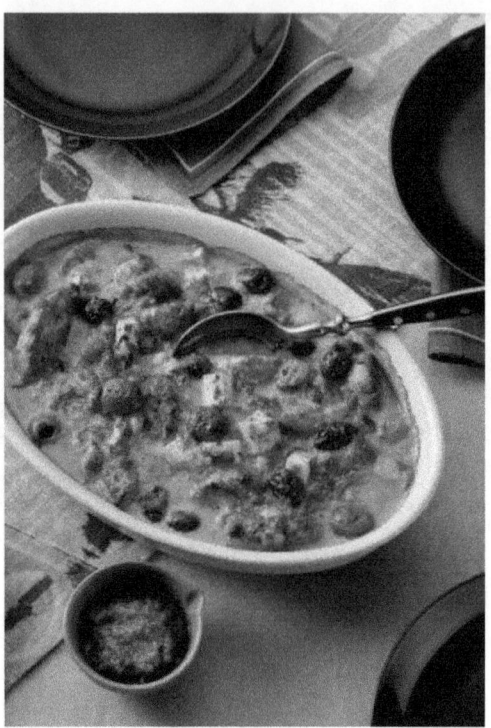

Ingredients

- 1 pound boneless, skinless chicken breast, cut into chunks
- 1 bunch fresh thyme sprigs
- 1 head cauliflower, cut into florets
- 1 shallot, finely chopped
- 3 tbsp. olive oil
- 1/2 tsp. sea salt
- 1 tsp. ground black pepper
- zest of 1 lemon
- 1/4 cup fresh lemon juice

- 1 cup olives, pitted
- 5 cloves garlic, thinly sliced

Directions

1. Spread thyme on the bottom of 7x11 baking dish. Place chicken over this and then distribute the cauliflower over the top.

2. In a separate bowl, combine remaining ingredients and mix thoroughly. Pour this mixture over the chicken but don't stir. Refrigerate at least one hour or preferably overnight.

3. Bake at 400F for 50 minutes, or until chicken is cooked through and cauliflower is browned and mixture is bubbling.

Makes 4 servings.

Asian Stir Fry

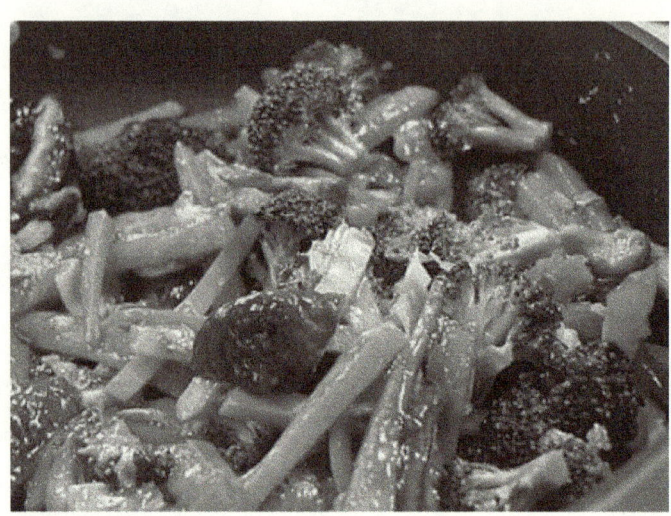

Ingredients

- 1 pound boneless, skinless chicken breast, cut into 1-inch cubes
- 2 tbsp. coconut oil
- 1 medium onion, peeled and finely chopped
- 2 heads broccoli, sliced
- 2 medium carrots, sliced
- 2 heads baby bok choy, sliced crosswise into strips
- 1 cup shiitake mushrooms, stemmed and thinly sliced
- 1 small zucchini, sliced
- 1/2 tsp. sea salt
- 1-1/2 cups water
- 2 tbsp. arrowroot powder
- 2 tbsp. toasted sesame oil
- 2 tbsp. plum vinegar

Directions

1. Heat coconut oil in large skillet and then sauté the onion for 10 minutes until soft. Add broccoli, carrots, and chicken, and sauté for another 10 minutes.

2. Add bok choy, mushrooms, zucchini, and salt, and cook for another 5 minutes. Add 1 cup of water, cover, and cook for 10 minutes, until vegetables are wilted.

3. In separate bowl, dissolve arrowroot powder in remaining 1/2 cup of water. Add to vegetable and chicken mix and cook for 2 minutes, stirring, until sauce thickens. Stir in sesame oil and vinegar and serve while still warm.

Makes 4 servings.

Don't forget to share your thoughts on this book by leaving a review on Amazon.com. It takes just a few seconds.

Zucchini Noodles

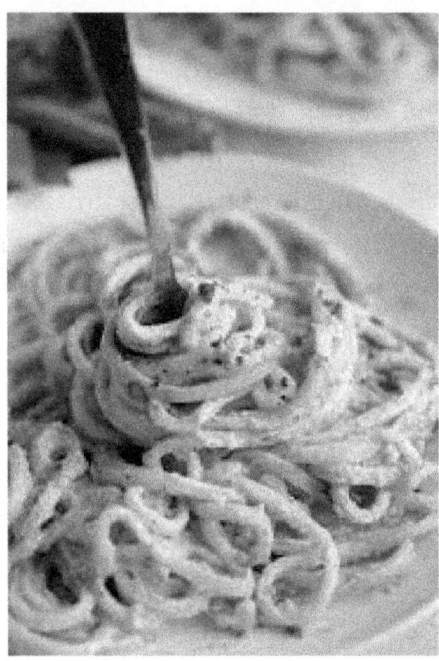

When you want the taste of noodles but can't find a low-carb option, these can be served on their own as a nice side dish or with a low-carb tomato sauce in place of pasta.

Ingredients

- 1 tbsp. olive oil
- 1 pound zucchini, shredded in long shreds (use a vegetable peeler for shredding zucchini)
- 1 tsp. all-purpose chef's shake, Italian seasoning, or another salt-free seasoning

Directions

1. Heat olive oil in large sauté pan. Add zucchini and seasoning and stir for 5 minutes, or until zucchini is tender.

2. Drain and serve, or noodles can be refrigerated and then reheated as needed.

Makes 4 servings.

Salmon Burgers

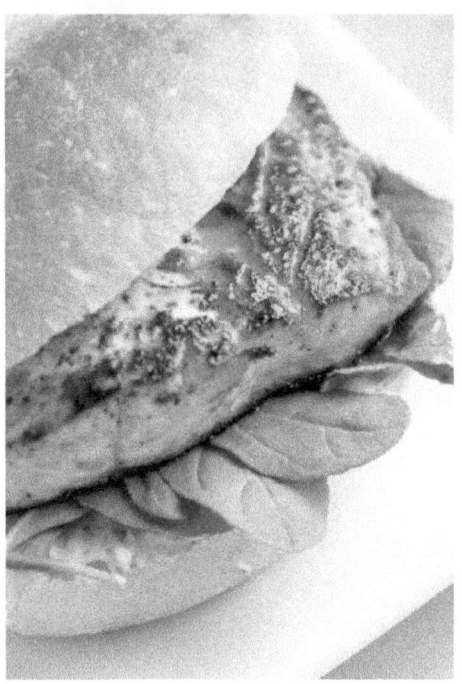

Ingredients

- 1 pound salmon, skin removed
- 1 tbsp. toasted sesame oil
- 1 tbsp. plum vinegar
- 1 clove garlic, pressed
- 1 tsp. minced ginger
- 1/4 cup chopped scallions
- 1/4 cup toasted sesame seeds
- 2 large eggs
- 1 tbsp. coconut flour
- coconut oil, for frying

Directions

1. Cut salmon into 1/4-inch cubes.

2. In large bowl, combine salmon with next 7 ingredients. Stir in flour. Form into 1/4-cup patties.

3. Heat coconut oil in large skillet and cook patties for about 5 minutes on each side, until golden brown. Transfer to paper towel to let drain for several seconds. Serve while still hot.

Makes 4 servings.

Ketogenic Brownies

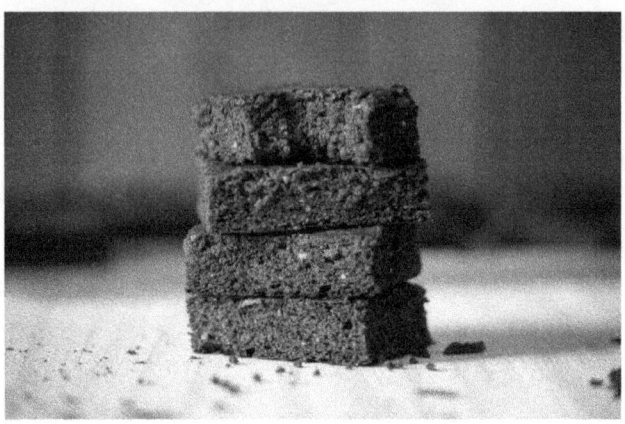

Ingredients

- 1 cup macadamia nuts
- 1/4 tsp. sea salt
- 1/4 tsp. baking soda
- 3 ounces 100% dark chocolate, chopped (lower percentage dark chocolate will have higher amounts of sugar so only use 100% dark)
- 1/2 cup coconut oil
- 2 tbsp. erythritol
- 3 large eggs
- 1 tsp. vanilla stevia sweetener

Directions

1. Use a food processor to pulse nuts, salt, and baking soda until coarse. Add in chocolate and coconut oil and continue to pulse until smooth.

2. Add remaining ingredients and pulse until consistency of brownie batter. Transfer to 8x8 baking dish and bake at 350F for 25 minutes. Allow to cool for at least one hour before serving.

Makes 16 brownies.

2-Ingredient Pudding

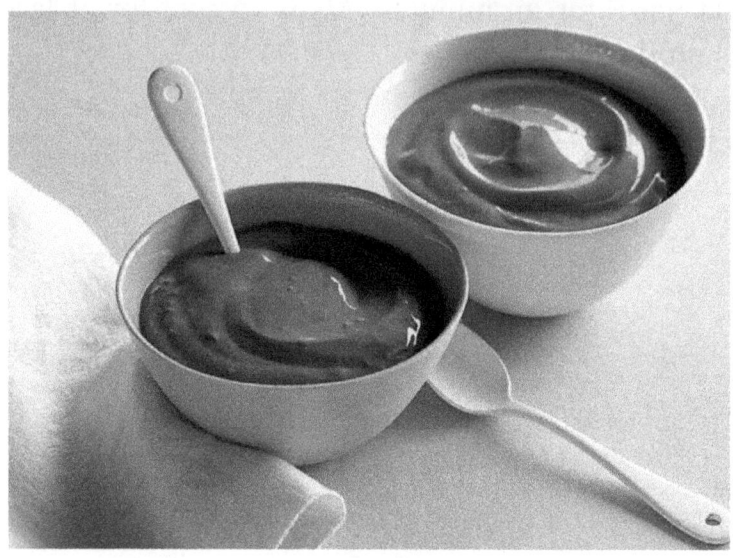

Ingredients

- 1 can coconut milk
- 1 cup chocolate chips

Directions

1. Heat coconut milk over very low heat and then add in chocolate. Stir constantly until chocolate is melted and is mixed thoroughly.

2. Dish into six individual 1/2-cup bowls, cups, or mason jars and refrigerate for at least 3 hours before serving.

Makes 6 servings.

Dark Rye Ketogenic Bread

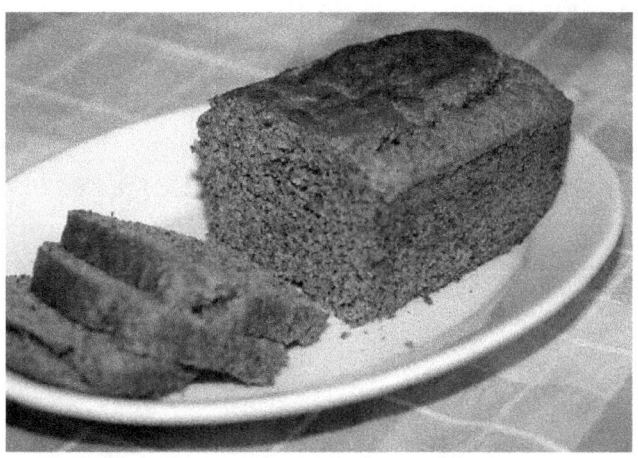

Ingredients

- 1 cup blanched almond flour (not almond meal)
- 3/4 cup brown flax meal
- 1/2 tsp. sea salt
- 1/2 tsp. baking soda
- 3/4 tsp. cream of tartar
- 3 large eggs
- 2 tbsp. olive oil
- 1/4 cup water
- 2 tbsp. caraway seeds

Directions

1. In one large mixing bowl, combine almond flour, flax meal, salt, baking soda, and cream of tartar; mix well and then set aside.

2. In separate bowl, combine eggs, oil, and water; mix thoroughly. Stir the wet ingredients into the dry ingredients and then add the seeds.

3. Mix, then leave batter for 2 minutes so it can thicken. Transfer to 7x3 loaf pan and bake at 350F for 40 minutes. Allow to cool for one hour before serving.

Makes one loaf.

Discover Scientifically-Proven "Shortcuts" & "Hacks" to Lose Weight FASTER (With Very Little Effort)

For this month only, you can get Linda's best-selling & most popular book absolutely free – *Weight Loss Secrets You NEED to Know.*

Get Your FREE Copy Here:
TopFitnessAdvice.com/Bonus

Discover scientifically-proven tips to help you lose weight faster and easier than ever before. With this book, readers were able to improve their weight loss results and fitness levels. So, it's highly recommended that you get this book, especially while it's free!

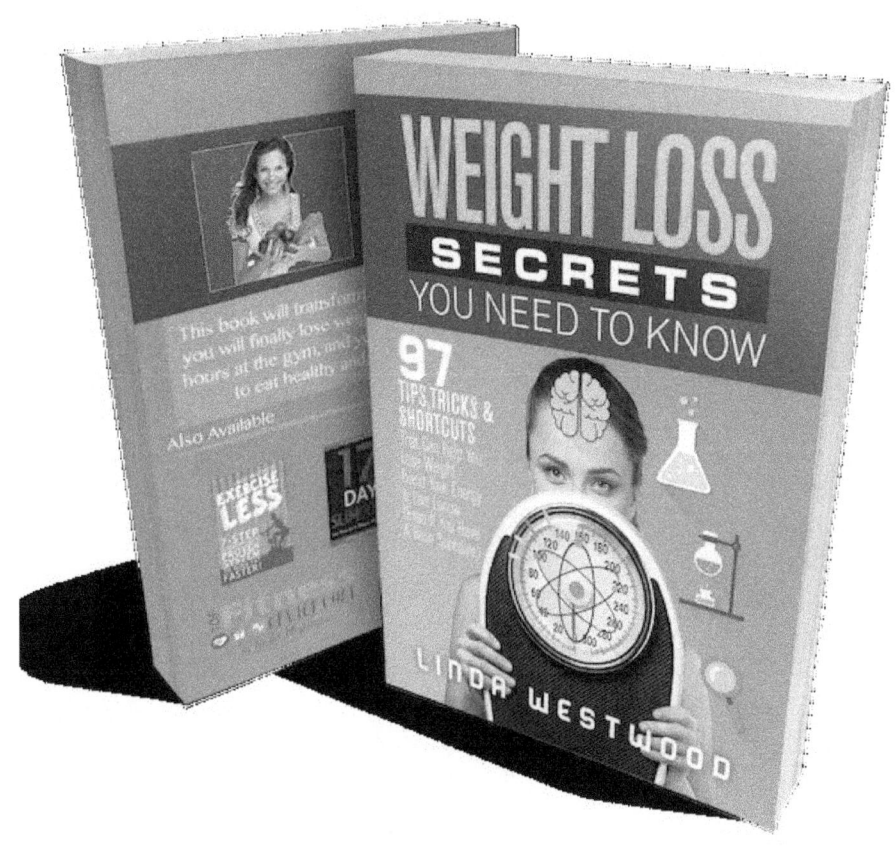

Get Your FREE Copy Here:
TopFitnessAdvice.com/Bonus

Conclusion

The ketogenic diet is a great way to watch pounds melt away, quickly and safely. Your own body turns into a fat burning machine, using up stores of fat rather than glucose from food you're eating for energy.

At the same time, it protects your heart and other muscles from damage since you're feeding them nourishing, healthy oils and lots of needed protein.

For the ketogenic diet to work, you don't need to necessarily count calories and weigh or measure your food, but as with all eating plans, you need to be honest with yourself about what you're eating and how much.

While virtually unlimited fats are allowed, it's good to get healthy, unsaturated fats that your body can easily digest and which won't clog your arteries; this means fats from fish, avocados, and peanuts, and olive oil. Lean protein choices are also better than fatty cuts of beef.

As with the rest of your food, you don't necessarily need to count carbohydrates, as long as you educate yourself about which foods are high in carbs and are sure to limit these in your diet.

If you do follow the ketogenic diet as recommended, you'll get a lean and toned physique in no time. You'll also calm your cravings, have a consistent source of energy, and won't feel fatigued throughout the day as you normally would.

If you're still not convinced that the ketogenic diet is for you, why not try it for a few weeks?

You have enough recipes in this book to prepare healthy and filling meals throughout the day and which will keep you full while also allowing your body to shift from burning glucose to burning fat.

In that short time, you might lose weight, gain energy, and find that the ketogenic diet is better than any you've ever tried before!

Final Words

I would like to thank you for purchasing my book and I hope I have been able to help you and educate you on something new.

If you have enjoyed this book and would like to share your positive thoughts, could you please take 30 seconds of your time to go back and give me a review on my Amazon book page.

I greatly appreciate seeing these reviews because it helps me share my hard work.

You can leave me a review on Amazon.com.

Again, thank you and I wish you all the best!

Enjoying this book?

Check out my other best sellers!

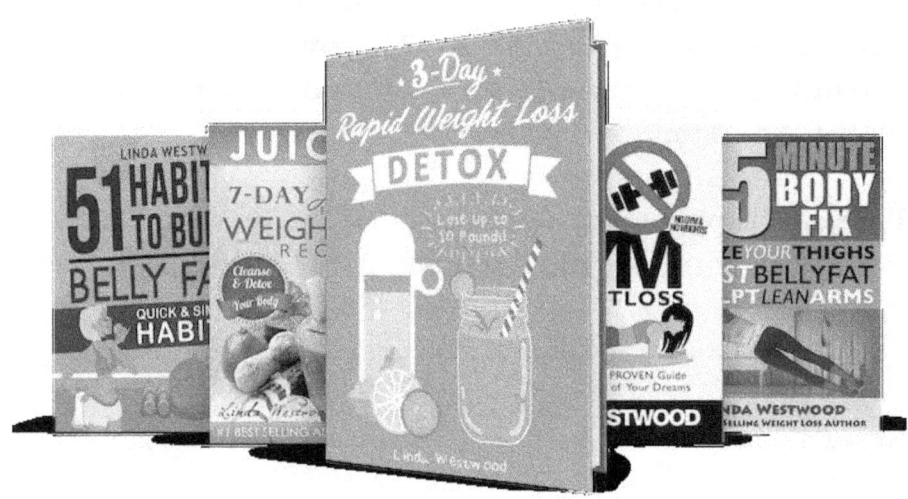

Get your next book on sale here:

TopFitnessAdvice.com/go/books

www.ingramcontent.com/pod-product-compliance
Lightning Source LLC
Chambersburg PA
CBHW031158020426
42333CB00013B/729